THE F WORD:
FIBROIDS, FEAR, AND THE FUTURE.

Kim Herring

Copyright © 2020 Kim Herring

All rights reserved. No part of this publication may be reproduced, distributed, or transmitted in any form or by any means, including photocopying, recording, or other electronic or mechanical methods, without the prior written permission of the publisher, except in the case of brief quotations embodied in critical reviews and certain other noncommercial uses permitted by copyright law.

Book Design by Aeysha

ACKNOWLEDGEMENTS

The Lord: for hearing me before I called You. For blessing me with Saraphina, my guardian angel of protection.

My Love: for relating to me in another dimension.

Grandmother: for your prayers and phone calls.

Mom: for your encouraging words early in the morning and your prayers.

TT: for texting me timely scriptures out of the blue.

Tony: for listening and letting me vent without judgement.

Harold: for giving me pep talks and reminding me that anything is possible.

Myisha and Traci: for sharing your children on video chat, I see you in them.

Jeana, Keturah, Lila, and Nisha: for answering my video chats when I cried, cussed, and spoke in circles.

Lashonde: My neighbor who turned into a forever friend by making sure I knew I was never alone.

Mar Ephrem and MTOC Fresno, Archbishop E. Bernard Jordan and Zoe Ministries, and Larry Reid Live: for your prayers, humor, and prophecies when I couldn't see the Light at the end of the tunnel.

Healing isn't linear and is almost always ugly, but it is necessary. My hope is that everyone who reads my words will connect in some way. Although our stories are not the same, there is a connectedness in crisis that help us know we are never alone in our experience.

PART ONE

I have an analytical brain, I do not like outliers. I like checkboxes and structures so whatever is being addressed has to make sense in order for me to process it. When that does not happen, my brain continues to run until it lands on the most likely scenario. As it relates to health, what makes sense to me and has made me feel the best in my body and brain is eating cleaner, being active, seeing my therapist, and keeping my spiritual life strong. Although not easy, it's the simplest way for me to feel safe and at peace with my own life. This way of living had proven beneficial to me for years. 2019 changed the game and my life would never be the same.

Chapter one

No matter the birth control method or how low the dose, my body did not react well to the hormones that were supposed to regulate me. Since my period only lasted 3 days, I didn't make a fuss and learned how to listen to my body for signs that the first day of my period was approaching. This worked well for me until January 2019. During my annual visit at the end of January, I told my then OBGYN my period was extremely heavy, lasted eight days, and had clots this month. She did the exam and after a few days called back to tell me there were no abnormalities found in my blood, all the tests were negative, and during the physical exam she didn't feel anything out of the ordinary. She told me to monitor myself for the next 3 months and let her know if anything has changed. As my OBGYN for the past 5 years, I didn't have any reason not to trust her medical opinion. She considered my age might have something to do with the change in my period because I was 43.

A few months later I went back to see my OBGYN because nothing had changed. She began asking me had I been stressed out or had I noticed any weight gain because these could be throwing my body out of sorts. I wasn't under any more significant stress and although I had gained a few pounds, I hadn't put on a 10lbs since my last visit. I asked for another physical exam and ultrasound.

I recall thinking that even if she did not feel anything from the physical exam, perhaps the ultrasound would show her something. Instead she talked about women going into early menopause at my age and that might be something I need to consider. Instead of the ultrasound, she recommended birth control because she did not feel anything abnormal with my second physical exam. Birth control, she said, would level the playing field if I gave it a chance, so I reluctantly agreed.

Mid-summer I returned and told her that I could no longer take birth control. As was my previous experience, the entire 3 months I used the birth control she prescribed, I had spotting and cramps. I remember only having 1 week a month where there was no spotting and no actual period. That's it, one week per month. During early fall, my period had returned to its original 3-day cycle! I was over the moon, I thought whatever was going on in my body worked itself out and things were back to normal. Until December rolled around and I spent the last 8 days of that month bleeding, nauseated, and depressed.

In January 2020, it was time for my annual again. I went back and told her it had been an entire year and we had tried all the diet changes, stress reduction tips, and birth control there was to try. The past few months on pill yielded nothing positive, because when I was not actually on my period, I was spotting. On this visit I asked her to do another exam and to do an ultrasound and that if she would not, I would be forced to go look for another provider because something was not right with my body. She gave me all her medical mumbo jumbo and financial reasons why she would not schedule the ultrasound, so I left.

Chapter two

I began looking for a new OBGYN on my approved provider list. Since my insurance provider would not pay for another annual by a new provider within the same year, the visit would be out of pocket, so I needed to save a few hundred dollars. By the time I saved the money and found the first two providers I wanted to schedule an appointment with, it was March and COVID-19 was here in full force. Since I was a new patient, both providers I chose scheduled my appointments for May because they were modifying their hours as well as cutting down on staff. Established patients were the priority so I had to wait.

One of the upcoming appointments with a new OBGYN had been cancelled. Apparently, the office spent the prior months transferring their existing patients to new providers in order to close down the practice. The other provider rescheduled me for June because they were still having challenges with limited staff. At this point COVID-19 had most things shut down in my state. Like many of you, I had been working out at home and learning new hobbies and skills via the internet. Pretty soon, those workouts were over before they began, and I didn't even bother logging on the computer to do anything outside of my 9-5. I had become extremely tired doing everyday things like cleaning my house and taking a shower. I would have to catch my breath before my warmups were even over. I am someone who used to jog/run and sing on a treadmill for 35 minutes, and now I had to take a break when I washed my hair. My annual physical was coming up in July and I knew I had to address this with my primary. I also intended on updating her on my OBGYN situation and asking for a referral.

I did not make it to my annual physical because on June 29,2020, I woke up in someone else's body. I opened my eyes to start my workday and an excruciating pain radiated through the lower right quadrant of my belly. I literally screamed and crawled out of the bed to get to the bathroom. I had no idea what was happening to me, but I knew I better get help fast. About an hour later, I was at the nearest Urgent Care facility. Thanks to COVID-19, nobody was there so I was called back no sooner than I filled out the paperwork.

The doctor asked what was going on and I explained what happened this morning as well as what had been happening with my period. The doctor lightly hit the back of my lower back and I just about jumped off the table. I did not know what she touched but when I turned back around to look at her she told me to go to an ER immediately. Not too far from the Urgent Care is my local hospital where again, no one was there except the receptionist, intake nurse, and myself. I was escorted back and put in a room where I put on the gown and awaited the blood tests. I eventually fell asleep but was startled awake by 3 nurses rushing in and asking me the date of my last transfusion. At the same time, another nurse asked me if I knew I was severely anemic to which I replied, "I absolutely did not know that." As they were preparing to give me a blood transfusion, the nurse asked me if I took an ambulance or did I have someone bring me to the ER and I told her that I drove from the Urgent Care directly here. The room stood still as a doctor said, "I'm not sure how you drove here, your hemoglobin is 6."

I received the blood transfusion then taken downstairs to have a CT of my abdomen. When I returned to the ER, I was told that not only was I severely anemic, but I also had a right kidney thrombosis and multiple uterine fibroids. Because of this, the hospital was preparing a room for me upstairs. I remember looking around the room in disbelief, shaking my head and saying, "wait a minute, what?"

Chapter three

I was inpatient 4 days, 3 of those days with a heparin drip in one arm and iron in the other. When I left the hospital, I went straight to my primary physician to begin a treatment plan. Dr. M. and I had been together for 5 years also and when I arrived, she was just as shocked as I was. I remember her pacing in the room while we talked about the 3 diagnoses I received. She could not believe I had these issues as I am one of her healthiest patients. She had the notes from all the providers and the vascular surgeon who saw me in the hospital and like them, she had no idea how all these things could be happening to me. We have noticed over our 5 years together, periods of low Vitamin D for me and we worked on my eating more grains and lentils but nothing remotely close to anemia or any signs of blood clots. She gave me a prescription for blood thinners, a referral to a hematologist, a new OBGYN that could see within 3 days, and an appointment for blood work the following week. Dr. M. was determined to get to the bottom of things if she could.

I used to feel confident and exited at doctors' offices because I was doing well but that changed. When the staff would call to remind me of an upcoming visit, I would get very anxious. Showing up to an appointment would ruin my entire day. The hematologist office the only space in the lower level of a building. When you got off the elevator, it was a large foyer that was dark and then you walk toward the double doors to enter the waiting room. I almost had a panic attack my first visit there. When I finally saw the hematologist and she asked what my history was I told her about my then OBGYN. As I told her the story, I began crying even though I tried not to. She told me, "well, sometimes we miss things, we are human" and I immediately dried the tears and shut down. (Sidenote, saying someone is human when they screw up is a pet peeve of mine.) I never spoke to her again about how I felt. She would ask how I felt because my eyes were puffy at each appointment and I would say I was fine. At each appointment, I would cry all the way to her office, stop when I arrived at her waiting room, and start back when I got to the elevator.

The OBGYN visits were no better. They were no better because each visit got progressively worse. The first I gave 9 vials of blood and had a quick physical exam where he told me he felt quite a few fibroids but wanted to get an ultrasound to confirm the amount. The next visit was more blood work and we talked about the options women have for fibroids including removing them, laparoscopic and abdominal hysterectomies. After the ultrasound, I had an MRI then went back to the OBGYN for a biopsy.

Let me tell you something, if the staff tells you it will feel like a pinch, do not believe them. It was the most excruciating 7 minutes I can recall in my entire life. The pain started as soon as the tool was inserted, and it did not end until well after the assistant turned the lights off and closed the door to let me cry and rest in peace. A week later I was told the news that would instantly devastate me. After reviewing the MRI, ultrasound, biopsy, and physical exam, it was determined I would need an abdominal partial hysterectomy with a 6-week recovery because the fibroids and my uterus were too big for any laparoscopic procedure.

My mind flashed back to 2019 when I first began talking to my then OBGYN about the ways my period had drastically changed, and she did nothing. Here I am, 43 years old being told I must have my stomach cut open to remove my womb. Could this have been avoided if my then OBGYN had taken me seriously the entire year of 2019? Would this be my fate had I been able to see a new OBGYN during the first quarter of 2020? How long had these things been growing? Why is everything so big? What the hell is going on here?

PART 2

This is where I want to start talking about how I have been processing the events from June 29th. From the minute I left that hospital admission, I no longer felt like myself, there was a sadness, an aloneness, and an anger present that was foreign to me. Since I am a creative person, I was using dance, song, writing, and art to flesh those emotions out. No matter what I drew, not matter what I wrote, the end result was a labyrinth with a hole in the center. I kept trying to figure out why this was happening to me and how? I ate clean, I worked out, I took the sea moss, elderberry, I drank ginger, turmeric tea, my spiritual life was strong, and I had a therapist. Other than being a Black woman there didn't seem to be any logical explanation for this.

Chapter one

While all this is happening, so is life in general. I now have to open an FMLA claim because I am going to multiple visits with multiple providers as well as an upcoming surgery. The company that handled my FMLA were the absolute worse. They denied every visit, which I had to appeal. Their appeal process required provider intervention which meant I had to sometimes go back to the provider for additional documentation. I would sit on the phone and explain my diagnoses and provider visits to this company so many times, that I recommended them to replay my previous calls since they are recorded. This is a company that touts the ease of reporting absences or provider visits on their website but that is not my experience.

I still work a full-time job, I am in school full time, and bills haven't stopped- in fact, they have increased because the bills related to June 29th are beginning to come in. I still have my family, my friends, and I wasn't always positive and present in all these areas even though the people in my life were present for me. They showed up for me, they blessed me, they prayed for me, but I still felt alone and scared. I wanted to talk to women who had my experience, so I began reading blogs and articles on women who have had abdominal hysterectomies. I had a few conversations with women who shared my same diagnoses and I honor them. What struck me is I didn't see my particular story and knew I had to tell my own story in my own way in my own time.

There were many women who had fibroids treated, before ever needing a hysterectomy. I found there were women who welcomed the procedure in order to alleviate the terrible symptoms they were living with. I found a remnant of women who were excited about the freedom a hysterectomy would bring by ending their period. My research was intense because I wasn't sleeping very well, an. I read about laparoscopic procedures, what people think causes fibroids, risk factors, and what you should look for in a surgeon. There is so much information out there, so many things to sort through but I found quite a few real-life experiences that I honor and take seriously. Those real-life experiences encouraged me to write this book.

Chapter two

In 2019, I wanted to have a child. Women are having children later in life and I knew I would more than likely need some sort of scientific help and started saving for it, especially since insurance covers little infertility costs. Once I found out my womb was going to be taken, the reality of never being a biological mother hit me like a ton of bricks. The entire year of advocating for myself to my then OBGYN felt like a year of failure on my part. I had so many questions but no answers. Why didn't I just leave after 3 months of her not doing anything? How long have these things been growing inside me? Is this happening because I have done something wrong or done someone wrong? Why didn't have kids in high school like everyone else?

Realizing that there will never be a human on this planet that I carried in my own body and birthed out is hard to talk to others about, but the questions and the feelings turned over in my mind constantly. I still see a mini-me running past me in my home, only to realize it is no longer it will remain a part of my imagination. I imagine what life would be like had I been able to carry and raise a little him or her. I was facing the finality of it all. I would never carry a child in my body. Not because I was too old, or didn't have enough money, or didn't have the right partner. I would never carry a child in my body because fibroids and late medical treatment stole the option from me.

Chapter three

I am emotionally overwhelmed and financially strapped. Angry and confused, I would talk to the recorder on my phone. I would talk about how angry I felt at what I called, aliens. How dare they invade my body and rip away my chance at motherhood? I have faced so many losses in life, from losing my father when I was 3 years old, to disconnecting from my partner due to mental illness, to everything in between. I couldn't understand how I was being forced to endure yet another loss. Have you ever had a punch to the gut? That is how I felt from the moment I found out about the aliens in my body and I recorded that multiple times a day. In therapy, we are taught not to use words like "never", or "always" when describing a person, but I was speaking about myself, to myself, and the word "never" kept rolling off my tongue. I had no space for toxic positivity, I was hurting and allowing myself to feel it all.

I have been using my savings and 401k to pay for many of the visits until my deductible kicked in. I had to pay for the ultrasound and both MRI's at the time of service. Once the deductible was met, I still had plenty to pay in coinsurance and balance bills. Deferring bills in order to pay out of pocket for medical challenges is a fact of life for many in the United States, and now I am one of the many. All of this financial weight and I haven't even had the surgery yet. Unless you are independently wealthy, getting sick in this country can literally cost you everything even with commercial insurance. Not only does it cost you financially, it costs you mentally and psychologically. This is trauma.

Surgery

I arrive for the surgery and feel like I have dissociated from my body. I feel very calm or numb, I can't tell which. Everything needs to be over and quick is all I keep thinking. I don't like the smell in the hospital, my gown, the socks, the heat blower they have on me, or anything else. It's nothing personal, I just don't want to be here and acutely aware of everything I dislike about my surroundings.

In the pre-op room, nurses and my surgeon are running in and out with questions and answers. The anesthesiologist comes to talk with me about her role in the surgery. She calmly explains that she will give me a cocktail of some sort once I enter the operating room and then give me the full experience of going under for surgery. We talk about how I will wake up in the post-op area, groggy but under observation until I am taken to my room to rest. When she has finished speaking, I ask what they are going to do with my womb. She is taken aback and replies that she has never been asked that question before. It was my turn to be shocked because I had been wondering about the final place of my womb since I was told it would be taken from me. It had been with me my whole life and I felt the need to know its final resting place. I was told my womb would be examined then considered medical waste to be incinerated. I didn't know I would need to unpack that at a later date.

When I woke up the next day and told I had to walk around, I felt like my insides were going to fall out. I walked to my bathroom, across the hall, then came back into my room and sat in the recliner. One of the doctors came in to see how I was feeling and was incredibly happy to know I had been walking and was now sitting in the chair. He let me know what a hard time they had removing my womb. Apparently, it had somehow burrowed itself deeper into my body causing challenges in its removal. In my mind I pictured it saying, "hell no, we won't go" and then I came back to earth to listen to him finish.

My uterus was:

- 19.5cm x 10.3cm x 12.5cm

The 4 fibroids were:

- 9.2cm x 7.4cm x7.1cm submucosal

- 6.0cm x 4.8cm x 4.4cm

- 4.1cm x 3.5cm x 2.5 submucosal

- 3.6cm x 3.5cm x2.5cm submucosal

Closing

72 hours later I was home preparing for my teletherapy visit. I was irritated, sad, uncomfortable, and angry. Dr. Karen pointed out that I was grieving an unexpected loss, possibly due to medical neglect. We discussed feeling my feelings without judgement, how to properly grieve, and finding a way to release the pain in a healthy manner. The best way I know how to do that is to create something, and this book you are holding is what I created.

As I write I know healing begins to take up space inside of me. I wrote every time I had big feelings but couldn't articulate them. I wrote hoping that someone would see themselves and know they aren't alone. I wrote to give a voice to the voiceless while amplifying my own. I wrote while tears fell down my cheeks and I wrote when I felt like God wasn't hearing me. I don't know what's on the other side of this book, but there is something. As I continue taking life day by day, I have no choice but to run into what's next, and when I do, I can't wait to share it.

www.ingramcontent.com/pod-product-compliance
Lightning Source LLC
Chambersburg PA
CBHW072210100526
44589CB00015B/2467